Pocket Manual on

The Art of History Taking

Pocket Manual on
The Art of History Taking

Third Edition

Shivananda Prabhu MS
Professor of Surgery
Kasturba Medical College
Mangalore, Karnataka, India

Foreword
BM Hegde

JAYPEE The Health Sciences Publisher
New Delhi | London | Philadelphia | Panama

Jaypee Brothers Medical Publishers (P) Ltd.

Headquarters

Jaypee Brothers Medical Publishers (P) Ltd.
4838/24, Ansari Road, Daryaganj
New Delhi 110 002, India
Phone: +91-11-43574357
Fax: +91-11-43574314
E-mail: jaypee@jaypeebrothers.com

Overseas Offices

J.P. Medical Ltd.
83, Victoria Street, London
SW1H 0HW (UK)
Phone: +44 20 3170 8910
Fax: +44 (0)20 3008 6180
E-mail: info@jpmedpub.com

Jaypee-Highlights Medical Publishers Inc.
City of Knowledge, Bld. 237, Clayton
Panama City, Panama
Phone: +1 507-301-0496
Fax: +1 507-301-0499
E-mail: cservice@jphmedical.com

Jaypee Medical Inc.
The Bourse
111, South Independence Mall East
Suite 835, Philadelphia, PA 19106, USA
Phone: +1 267-519-9789
E-mail: jpmed.us@gmail.com

Jaypee Brothers Medical Publishers (P) Ltd.
17/1-B, Babar Road, Block-B, Shaymali
Mohammadpur, Dhaka-1207
Bangladesh
Mobile: +08801912003485
E-mail: jaypeedhaka@gmail.com

Jaypee Brothers Medical Publishers (P) Ltd.
Bhotahity, Kathmandu, Nepal
Phone: +977-9741283608
E-mail: Kathmandu@jaypeebrothers.com

Website: www.jaypeebrothers.com
Website: www.jaypeedigital.com

Inquiries for bulk sales may be solicited at: jaypee@jaypeebrothers.com

Pocket Manual on the Art of History Taking

First Edition: 2004

Second Edition: 2009

Third Edition: **2015**

ISBN: 978-93-5152-625-4

Printed at Rajkamal Electric Press, Plot No. 2, Phase-IV, Kundli, Haryana.

Dedicated to

My wife Mamatha

and

Son Samarth

whose affection is my strength

Foreword

If you listen to your patient long enough,
he/she will tell you what is wrong with him/her.

— Lord Platt, 1949

Listening to patients' joys and sorrows is itself an art. Henry David Thoreau wrote, "To affect the quality of the day—that is the highest of arts." Medicine has the capacity to affect the quality of the human day. The art of history taking is that which improves the quality of the day for the patient. To test the relevance of Platt's statement of 1949, five of Platt's students carried out a new double blind, computerized, prospective study on one hundred outpatients in London teaching hospitals. The results were an eye opener. Eighty per cent of the accurate final diagnosis and one hundred per cent of the future management strategies could be chalked out at the end of reading the referral letter and **listening** to the patient. This figure was slightly improved by four per cent by all kinds of bedside physical examinations and eight more per cent by every single investigation right up to positron emission tomography! This speaks volumes about the strength of listening to the patient carefully, which is otherwise called history taking. We shall stick to the word listening in this foreword.

Listening is a difficult art and has to be mastered by a humane doctor who has an insight into another's problems. Although we could teach students all about history taking, each physician, in his own life, learns the tricks of the trade as listening cannot be straight jacketed into watertight compartments. The rules of the game vary depending on the players. It is very easy to talk to someone but very difficult to listen to another's problems. The most important clue to listening is to give one's undivided attention to everything that the patient wants to tell. That said, I must hasten to add that some patients could be difficult candidates for this part of the clinical assessment as they talk twenty to a dozen and most of it is irrelevant. It is here that a master clinician scores over the mundane. The former would have evolved his/her own strategy to separate the wheat from the chaff in such long winded dialogues! That is called the wisdom which uses the knowledge one acquires from books and journals to evolve one's own style and learns everyday to fine tune the art of listening.

Dr Shivananda Prabhu, an erstwhile colleague of mine, our Professor of Surgery, has done a commendable job in this very difficult field. He reminds me of a Western plastic surgeon, Prof Calnan, who had written his classic *Talking with Patients* some years ago. Surgeons need to listen to patients more than physicians if they want to command the confidence of the patient. Talking with patients simply means listening to patients. It is not talking to patients. Dr Shivananda Prabhu has done well and I am sure he has succeeded in his efforts. Our patients cannot be assessed according to Western standards. History taking involves many imponderables—patient's educational background, his economic status, his religious and cultural ethos, his family values, his past experience with the medical profession, as also, his state of mind. That apart, every patient is very comfortable in his own mother tongue to express his heart's desires and longings. Working knowledge of patient's own language could be an added asset to the clinician.

I enjoyed going through this book and feel that this is an essential addition to the plethora of books that medical students have to cope with these days. This could be a clinical companion to every student, budding clinicians and, even to experienced clinicians to refresh their memory. I shall be happy to see it in every doctor's library. While I wish the author good luck, I hope this book will last long as this "art" of medicine does not change as fast as the so-called science of medicine does. Consequently, this book will have a longer shelf life. The get up of the book and the printing is excellent. The language of the book is very readable as it flows smoothly and is very lucid in its style. Overall, this book gets very high marks in my assessment. I recommend it very strongly.

"I do not know a better training for a writer than to spend some years in the medical profession—the doctor, especially the hospital doctor, sees human nature bare."

Somerset Maugham in THE SUMMING UP (1938)

(Maugham was trained as a physician at St Thomas' Hospital, London where seventy years earlier, John Keats was trained).

"Manjunath"
Pais Hills, Bejai
Mangalore-575 004
Karnataka, India

BM Hegde
MD FRCP (Lond) FRCP (Edinb)
FRCP (Glasg) FRCPI
FACC (USA) FAMS
Visiting Professor of Cardiology
University of London
Former Vice Chancellor
MAHE Deemed University
Ex-Director-Professor and Dean
Kasturba Medical College
Mangalore, Karnataka, India

Preface to the Third Edition

I am happy to note that *Pocket Manual on The Art of History Taking* has retained its popularity and is currently in its 3rd edition.

The need for a good book on the subject of history taking is a constant even in today's technology-driven world. This edition has retained its emphasis on principle rather than the technique of history taking. In addition, it has a separate chapter on the "Impediments to Good History Taking", which need to be understood by all concerned before they can be resolved. I believe, it will be useful to students as well as administrators of busy hospitals.

It would be failing in my duty if I do not express my deep appreciation and heartfelt gratitude to M/s Jaypee Brothers Medical Publishers (P) Ltd, New Delhi, India, for their constant support as well as encouragement. I am sure their diligence will ensure enthusiastic response from the student community.

Shivananda Prabhu

Preface to the First Edition

Medical Science has indeed progressed by leaps and bounds in the last few decades. Many diseases whose presence could only have been guessed in the days gone by can now be diagnosed accurately owing to the availability of newer investigative tools. Unfortunately, technological advance can be a double-edged sword. While one can definitely argue that this has made a clinician's job easier, it has given the clinician a false sense of security. I have been witness to a trend amongst medical fraternity to emphasise the investigative aspect of the clinical case discussion more than history taking or clinical examination. After all, one is going to need a CT scan or an MRI anyway to diagnose the condition; so why bother with detailed history taking and clinical examination is the usual argument in favour of the new trend. Well, this is a pathetic trend that needs no emphasis; and dangerous too.

William Osler's famous statement is worth reproducing here:

"To study the phenomenon of disease without books is to sail an uncharted sea, while to study books without patients is not to go to sea at all."

The foregoing altruism is enough evidence that the patient is indeed the centre of medical universe. If that is accepted, then how can we even contemplate reducing him to the status of a lab animal? Should we not hear his side of the story first? An anxious patient who walks into the outpatient clinic would like nothing worse than being asked to get a list of tests done straight away. He would surely like his doctor to hear him first, talk to him next, then examine him and finally ask for tests only if necessary. A doctor's sympathetic words mean as much to the patient as his treatment or even more sometimes. Many patients need only soothing words and not drugs to cure them. When one realises that in today's world it is the stress related and psychosomatic and not the organic diseases that haunt the mankind, the importance of proper communication becomes crystal clear. It is this "art of talking" that is dying today. It is my nightmare that one day outpatient clinics will be managed not by the clinicians but by a computer asking the patient to answer a questionnaire, drawing blood for investigations and scanning the patient all at the same time. I am sure you agree with me that it will be a sad day. What you are going to read in this book is my effort at preventing the species called Clinician from becoming extinct.

Well, one might legitimately ask me why clinical examination has not been discussed in this book. Normally thorough history taking should be followed by detailed clinical examination, both processes accomplished without any preconceived ideas about the diagnosis. Subjective information gleaned from the patient's history analysed together with the objective evidence got from clinical examination would ordinarily lead the clinician to the correct diagnosis or at least fairly close to it. Well, why then have I not discussed clinical examination methods in this book? The answer is very simple. Already there are excellent manuals on techniques of clinical examination, written by both Indian and Foreign authors, available to us. It will be pretty difficult for anybody to improve upon the exquisite details that some of these books give about the various techniques of clinical examination. And, they have the assistance of high-quality clinical photographs too. Unfortunately, while they demonstrate the necessary clinical skills elegantly, they often do not go beyond the routine on the matter of history taking. Perhaps in their effort to limit the size of the manual to manageable proportions history taking was not given its due importance by the authors. Hence, while the student of clinical surgery has ready access to excellent manuals of techniques of examination, the art of history taking remains by and large ignored. It is with this scenario in mind that I have avoided discussing details of techniques of examination. My effort is to encourage the aspiring clinician to learn the art of communication first. Technique will follow.

It is my firm belief that without acquiring a level of skill in the art of history taking, one's clinical acumen is likely to stagnate. A good history will not only help in establishing a rapport with the patient but can also guide both clinical examination and investigations. It is only natural that I would discuss history taking in a surgical setting from a surgeon's point of view. While I am aware that it may not be the only point of view in a given situation, it is not a bad way to start your journey towards perfection, if such a thing exists! This book is meant for residents working in surgery wards. If others too find it useful, I will feel honoured.

As my endeavour is to encourage students of surgery to think for themselves, I have made no attempt to go into all individual symptoms pertaining to different diseases. A brief outline of how to develop an informative history based on what the patient says is given. These guidelines are generally applicable to all cases irrespective of the organ of origin of the disease process. Specific details regarding symptomatology, if needed, may please be had from more voluminous books.

As is clear from the foregoing paragraph, this book is not meant to be an alternative to existing clinical manuals but is meant to complement them. By itself it may not take the student of surgery very far, but it will add value to the information given in the clinical manual or perhaps make the students appreciate such information better.

What you are going to read is the fruit of my experience in the surgical wards over the years. I have learnt from my teachers as well as my students. I have also learnt from my own mistakes. I hope students also learn from my mistakes and not wait to commit their own. He is a wise man who learns from the mistakes committed by others. If the reader finds this book's approach to history taking novel and useful, the credit goes to my teachers, colleagues and dear students. The drawbacks, if any, on the other hand, will entirely be mine.

I might have referred to the patient as 'he' at most places. Such political incorrectness may be excused and 'he' may be taken to mean she at most such places, with obvious exceptions.

I conclude by expressing my sincere gratitude to Professor BM Hegde, a towering personality in his chosen field. The kind words he has said in his foreword to the book will continue to encourage me all my life. I only hope the rest of the book lives up to the standards set by Professor Hegde in his brilliant foreword.

Shivananda Prabhu

Contents

1

The Art of History Taking

WHY IS IT AN ART AND NOT MERELY A SCIENCE?

Well, history taking is an art simply because you can never be perfect in it. In any art, perfection can only be an ideal. One can only work towards it without ever achieving it. An artist, in the strictest sense will always be a student. Also an art cannot exactly be taught. Different people perceive it differently. It is for the interested individual to persue and learn the art himself. The same holds good when pursuing the art of history taking.

Medical students working in the wards should keep their eyes and ears open all the time and be constantly on the lookout for useful bits of information coming from any source. A pearl of wisdom might come forth from an experienced teacher at any time and not be repeated again. Such bits of common sense might come forth even from the ward nurse or the patient himself. If the student latches on to all such information that comes his way, in time a rich and highly useful bank of clinical information will be at his/her disposal. This will assist the student in gaining new insight into the patient's predicament.

History taking can never be mastered by anybody without being able to speak the patient's language. In fact, history taking involves the art of communication as well. Communication is well nigh impossible if there is a language barrier. Hence, a medical student working in the ward should make every effort to learn the local language. For example, there is no excuse for a student from a Hindi speaking state not knowing Kannada if he is studying in Bangalore and *vice versa*. Using a translator can only be a temporary arrangement. Unfortunately, I have seen students going through the whole medical course without learning even bits of the local language. Perhaps this is a sign of the times we live in where standards expected are being lowered all the time. I am afraid their time in the wards was simply wasted. On the other hand, there is no point expecting the patient to learn doctor's language. It will never happen. The mountain does not come to Muhmad!

Last but not least, one should provide adequate privacy in the examination room for the patient to feel comfortable and be able to come out with details of his trouble and innermost anxieties. The quality of history taken in a crowded and noisy outpatient clinic is not likely to be of the highest order.

Once you have the right attitude and the necessary linguistic as well as communicative skills you are on your way to be the maestro. It is not easy to be able to collect a good history. But I can assure you that the satisfaction that comes out of being able to take a good history and thus help in making an accurate diagnosis will more than compensate for the effort put in.

I have a small piece of advice before proceeding to history proper. It is said " Common sense in an uncommon degree is what the world calls wisdom". Apply your common sense at every step and you will slowly find out that clinical surgery is nothing but collection of small bits of common sense applied judiciously. In surgery most of the disease processes occur at a macro level and affect an anatomical organ that can easily be visualised. An adequate knowledge of the functional anatomy of particular organ will enable the clinician to visualise the symptoms the disease affecting it is likely to produce. Such knowledge is definitely the forerunner of a well taken history. I will not be surprised if after reading this book you feel that you already knew every bit of what is written in this book. It is then only a case of practising what we already know. That should not be too difficult. Come on, lets get started.

2

Preliminary Information About the Patient

Preliminary information refers to the details regarding patient's age, sex, religion, residential address, occupation, etc. Most of us routinely note down these facts. Many a time these details are already entered into the case file either by the billing clerk or by the nurse before the patient meets his doctor. We rarely pause to ponder over these data as we are usually impatient to hear the patient's complaints. Hence, let us first find out why these details about the patient need be collected personally and how they can direct the line of questioning occasionally.

One should always note down a patient's full name. It helps to establish an immediate rapport with the patient. The significance of doctor-patient relationship is too great to require emphasis here. Imagine a patient waiting in the ward for morning rounds by the consultant. He will obviously be physically infirm and emotionally insecure. And then the consultant comes and asks him sympathetically " how are you today, Mr Shetty?" It will have a two-fold effect on Mr Shetty, the patient. One is that he feels emotionally reassured that his doctor remembers him and hence likely to take care of his health. And the other is that he can narrate his worries or symptoms without hesitation, now that he has been invited to talk.

A seemingly minor gesture on the part of the clinician, but the effect on the patient is immense.

Many a time while working in the wards we heartlessly refer to patient's as 'cases'. We often ask things like "how is yesterday's hernia case doing ?" "When is the hydrocele case being discharged ?" and so on. At times we do not even acknowledge the patient's presence while discussing the details of the case in front of him. All this is nothing but dehumanising the patient. A patient would like to be treated with respect, if not with love and affection. Put yourself in the patient's place and you will never call him a case again.

Also, knowing a patient's name might give a clue to the patient's religious faith and thus his social customs and dietary habits. Often the surname part of a patient's name will provide a good indication as to which part of India he/she hails from, e.g. A Mr Nair is likely to be from Kerala, whereas Mr Shinde is from Maharashtra, India. This piece of information will help in suspecting endemic diseases prevalent in those regions especially when one is working in a tertiary care hospital catering to a large part of the country.

Age and sex are to be recorded routinely as they might indicate the possible pathology affecting the patient. Though one can guess a patient's age just by looking at him, such guesstimates are not always accurate and should be avoided. Many diseases are age related, e.g. children are more likely to suffer from congenital conditions, malnutrition, gastroenteritis, viral diseases, skin and soft tissue infection, etc. In young adults active tuberculosis, accident and trauma, psychosomatic illness, sexually transmitted conditions, etc. are more common than in other age groups. Middle aged persons might suffer from diabetes, chronic lung conditions, coronary artery disease, etc. And elderly people are prone for malignancy, degenerative diseases, malnutrition, etc. A more comprehensive list of diseases affecting different age groups is given at the end of this chapter. This list is by no means exhaustive and should never be relied on for anything more than initial suspicion regarding the possible pathology. After all, diseases do not read textbooks and have a nasty habit of affecting all age groups to a lesser or greater degree. Hence, age alone should not be used to include or exclude any pathology as a possibility.

Recording the patient's sex may seem superfluous on most occasions as the fact is obvious at sight. But it may not always be so, especially in very young children and grossly emaciated and bedridden patients. It is always a good policy to get the fact clarified if there is any doubt. Thus you will save yourself from acute embarrassment flowing out of ignorant assumptions. As is well known, many diseases are more common in females like thyroid disorders, varicose veins, functional disorders, etc. One need not stress that gynaecological conditions often present in surgical OPD as acute abdominal pain thus complicating the picture. Similarly certain other conditions like oropharyngeal malignancies, cirrhosis of the liver, peripheral vascular disease, etc. are more common in men. Again a list of diseases more common in either gender is given at the end of the chapter.

Everybody knows why a patient's address has to be recorded. It helps to inform the relatives in case of an emergency and also gives a clue to the probable endemic diseases prevalent in the area of patient's residence. But unfortunately knowledge does not always get translated into practice. It is only when one tries to contact the patient after his discharge from the hospital that one finds out how inadequately the address had been recorded. Hence, patient's full residential address along with the telephone number should ideally be recorded in the case sheet.

Somehow we have all been taught to ask about patient's occupation in the same breath as his address. There is nothing inherently wrong with such a policy, but it is likely that the due importance is not given to it by the students at this stage, as they will be anxious to start with the history of presenting complaints. One cannot afford to overlook this important aspect of patient's history which might indeed be the source of his problems. Hence, it is necessary to ask the details of occupation as a separate entity later in the history.

Pointed questions regarding patient's religion may not be considered polite by many. It is indeed so. But occasionally religion tends to dictate lifestyle. For example, some religions like Jainism strictly prohibit non-vegetarian food. Hence, the quality of diet will change. Sometimes faith controls the behaviour of the patient too, e.g. Jehovah's witnesses do not accept blood transfusions and organ transplants as a matter of faith. Unless it is absolutely unavoidable, one should try not to offend the patient's religious sensibilities. Replacing faith with logic is not always easy and should not be tried without a good reason.

Many a time the preliminary data collected is read out in a disjointed manner by the student presenting the case for discussion, e.g. "Ramappa, male 62 years, occupation farmer, resides in Mangalore." Does not it sound jarring? Now listen to this "Mr Ramappa, 62-year-old farmer, residing in Mangalore has the following complaints". The second statement contains the same information but is streamlined and has a nice ring to it. Well begun is half done as they say.

Occasionally patient himself may not be able to give the history for a variety of reasons-poor general condition, deaf-mutism, etc. Also when the patient is a very young child or is mentally retarded history will have to be taken from a relative or the person accompanying the patient. In all such cases it is necessary to record the name of such person and his relationship with the patient.

Remember that history has to be recorded in the same way that it is told by the patient. In other words, using layman's language. For example, if a person gives history of passing stools admixed with blood it should be recorded the same way in the history sheet and not as haematochezia.

DISEASE MORE COMMON IN MEN (EXCLUDING DISEASES OF THE GENITALIA)

- Malignancies of the upper aerodigestive tract
- Peripheral vascular disease like Buerger's disease and atherosclerosis
- Inguinal hernia
- Acid peptic disease
- Pilonidal sinus
- Haemophilia
- Cirrhosis of the liver

- Trauma
- Hodgkin's lymphoma
- Adenolymphoma
- Congenital hypertrophic pyloric stenosis
- Pharyngeal pouch (Students are encouraged to add to this list).

DISEASES MORE COMMON IN WOMEN (EXCLUDING DISEASES INVOLVING GENITALIA)

- All thyroid disorders
- Gallstone disease
- Femoral hernia
- Cushing's syndrome
- Urinary tract infection
- Raynaud's disease
- Hiatus hernia
- Rectal prolapse
- Idiopathic thrombocytopenic purpura
- Functional disorders
- Melanoma
- Carpal tunnel syndrome
- Keloid
- Desmoid tumour
- Erythrocyanotic (Bazin's) ulcer.

DISEASES COMMON IN CHILDREN

- All congenital abnormalities including malformations, embryological aberrations and genetic disorders

- Tumours like neuroblastoma, Wilms' tumours, Burkitt's lymphoma, leukaemias, etc.
- Skin and soft tissue infections
- Middle ear infections
- Ingestion of foreign bodies.

DISEASES COMMON IN ELDERLY

- Most malignancies, especially carcinoma of breast in women
- Benign prostatic hypertrophy in men
- Atherosclerosis and related cardiovascular problems
- Diabetes and it's long-term complications
- Malnourishment and asthenia
- Constipation
- Loneliness and other emotional problems
- Osteoarthritis
- Senile cataract
- Alzheimer's disease and other cerebral disorders of senescence.

3

Chief Complaints and History of Presenting Illness

Well, we have now come to the most important part of the history taking. A patient's history is indeed "his story". This story begins when the patient first experiences any of the symptoms which ultimately bring him to the hospital and leads right up to that day on which history is being taken. It is necessary to remember that history taking does not end with the patient getting admitted to the hospital. Many times a patient will have been in the hospital for weeks before the student gets to examine him. Indeed, he will have undergone tests and investigations about which he may tell you, if asked. These details may throw light on the probable diagnosis.

It is expected by now, one will have established a working relationship with the patient. Not too many patients enjoy being interviewed and examined repeatedly, least of all by beginners. It is indeed a delicate situation. The patient should be reassured that his predicament is understood by you and that you will do your utmost to make him comfortable. Of course, your actions should reflect your concern. Patient's sensibilities will have to be respected and anything that might cause pain either physical or emotional should be avoided, if at all possible. Questions related to patient's personal or marital life should be phrased carefully to avoid embarrassment.

The most important thing to remember while taking history is that the patient may not tell you the full story. He or she will have their reasons for suppressing parts of history. For example, the patient may not be very intelligent and hence may not understand your question fully. He might just tell you the symptom that bothers him most and keep quiet. This requires rephrasing the question in simpler terms. Remember, it is the less intelligent patients who test your history taking skills and not the intelligent ones. Remember also that occasionally patients might not reveal some facts are as they are embarrassed or think those facts are irrelevant. Some patients might have gone to other doctors before seeing you and may not reveal it as they feel it might offend you. It is up to the watchful clinician to ferret out all such useful information that the patient might have. Others may suppress some facts as they fear that if they tell everything they will be diagnosed to have a serious disease! At the other end of the spectrum are malingerers and oversmart patients who knowingly give false history. These are usually patients who want to shirk work and hence are looking for a gullible doctor to get a medical illness certificate. Well, sickness absenteeism is already a problem plaguing the economy of the country. Try not to add to it! With experience, it will be possible to spot them as their history will not conform to any known disease pattern. And of course, there will be an occasional patient who genuinely believes he has a problem in spite of not having any. In the face of such varied patient profile a clinician has to wear a detective's hat also, from time-to-time.

How do we start collecting history then? You can start by simply asking questions like "Mr Ramappa, what bring you to the hospital?" or "what can I do for you?" He will then start listing his complaints. Make the patient comfortable by requesting him to sit. Encourage him to start from the beginning and proceed from there, chronologically listing all complaints. Initially it is better not to interrupt his talk unless he goes too far off the track. Just encourage him by an occasional remark like "Okay, then what happened?" etc. Thus encouraged, a patient might reveal his inner most fears and anxieties apart from the physical symptoms. During this process if the clinician wants to get a certain point clarified he can do so by asking a direct but simple question, e.g.' What happened to the pain after you took the medication?' Try not to ask leading questions. Leading questions are those which imply the answer and force the patient to answer in 'Yes' or 'No'. They might simply choose 'yes' or 'no' depending on what they think will please the doctor. For example, if we were to rephrase the earlier question as "the pain reduced after taking the medication, didn't it ?" makes it a leading question.

Often, we are under the mistaken impression that the presenting history has to be of relatively short duration. Not so. For example, a person suffering from ureteric colic might have a duration of symptoms of few hours whereas a patient of ulcerative colitis might have been suffering without a break for years. In conclusion, the whole period for which the patient has been suffering from a particular symptom without a break should be included in the presenting history. That means presenting history starts at that point in the patient's past when he was apparently healthy for the last time. For example, "Patient was apparently healthy 6 months back, when a swelling appeared insidiously in the left axilla" and so on. On the other hand, if the patient has had multiple episodes of particular symptom with periods of complete normalcy in between them, then only the current episode becomes part of the presenting history. The previous episodes should then be included as part of the past history.

At the end of this process, clinician should have enough information to answer the following questions regarding each symptom.

1. When it started, i.e. the duration of the particular symptom?

If the patient has more than one symptom they should be noted down in the history sheet in the chronological order. For example,

- Upper abdominal pain—6 months
- Bloating sensation—4 months
- Vomiting—1 month

If two symptoms have appeared around the same time then the more specific or important of the two, as perceived by the clinician should be noted first. For example,

Jaundice—15 days
Loss of appetite—15 days

Here jaundice has been mentioned as the first symptom as it is more specific of the two.

This initial recording of "chief complaints" helps in streamlining the course of history taking.

2. How it started, i.e. the mode of onset?

Onset can be acute or insidious. "Acute onset" refers to a symptom which becomes fully manifest within a period of few hours to few days at the most. Insidious onset is that which takes a few days to one or two weeks to manifest fully. In case of a swelling note whether the duration refers to the swelling actually starting or the patient noticing the swelling. If the patient had merely noticed a swelling at a particular point of time it is possible that the swelling was there for quite some time before that. It is important to know whether the onset of a symptom was associated with any specific event, e.g. trauma, ingestion of particular food or medicine. It can give a clue to the probable diagnosis, e.g. a swelling which follows trauma could be a haematoma. Similarly pain abdomen following ingestion of analgesic is likely to be due to gastritis. Occasionally patients give history of minor trauma associated with the onset of swelling, e.g. hydrocele. Here it is likely that the swelling was already present and the trauma merely drew patient's attention to the swelling.

3. What is the nature of symptom?

The exact nature or specific characteristics of the symptom should be ascertained. This will help the clinician in understanding the underlying pathology. It is natural that only important symptoms caused by common surgical problems have been discussed briefly. Further details can be had from more elaborate clinical manuals.

- *Pain:* Pain is the most common symptom that makes the patient come to the hospital. We have been taught traditionally that pain could be of several types—burning, throbbing, stabbing, griping, boring, gnawing and so on. But in reality most patients find it difficult to express the exact nature of pain in words, though burning pain of acid peptic disease and throbbing pain of an abscess are useful clues to the diagnosis if the patient expresses the nature of pain clearly. One should not overly depend on it. There are two aspects of pain that any patient can understand—whether the pain is continuous or episodic and whether he would consider the pain severe in degree or not. Colicky pain suggests obstruction to a hollow tubular organ (e.g. intestinal obstruction, biliary colic, ureteric colic) while constant continuous pain indicates on going inflammation (e.g. acute pancreatitis) or ischaemia (e.g. mesenteric infarction). It is possible that what was initially a colicky pain might later change character into a continuous ache. These two aspects of pain, if clarified by the patient are often enough to indicate the pathological process causing the pain when analysed together with other data in the history.

Pain can be visceral or somatic depending upon the organ of origin and the type of nerve supply. The localization of the site of somatic pain is specific while the visceral pain is poorly localized. Hence, it should not be too difficult to identify the organ of origin of somatic or superficial pain, e.g. subcutaneous abscess, haematoma, etc. But visceral pain originating from intraperitoneal organs is ill localised early on. In the early postoperative period one has to be careful not to miss a visceral pain which might be masked by the somatic pain originating from the operative wound.

An interesting aspect of visceral pain which should be looked into by the clinician is whether the pain either radiates or is referred to any other site. Pain is occasionally referred to a site anatomically discontinuous from the organ of origin of the pain. This is due to the same segmental nerve roots supplying both the sites. For example diaphragmatic irritation due to blood, pus, etc. might result in the pain getting referred to the ipsilateral shoulder tip as both phrenic nerve and supraclavicular nerves share the same nerve roots (C4). Pain impulse is initially carried by the phrenic nerve and then gets referred to the shoulder tip and neck regions which share the same sensory supply. Similarly pain originating from the biliary tract might be referred to interscapular region (T 7-9). (Boas' sign). Pain of ureteric colic is often referred to the testicle(L1,2) on the same side.

On the other hand, radiation of pain means the spread of pain in a continuous manner to an adjacent organ while the original pain persists, e.g. the epigastric and left hypochondrial pain of pancreatitis radiating to the back. Loin to groin radiation of pain in ureteric colic is another classical example. Radiation of pain is usually due to the spread of pathological process or involvement of an adjacent organ. This has to be differentiated from "migration" of pain from one site to another, e.g. the periumbilical pain felt initially in acute appendicitis later migrates to right iliac fossa. This is due to a change in the mechanism of origin of pain from visceral to somatic.

Causes for Colicky or Episodic Pain

- **Acute intestinal obstruction due to a mechanical cause:** Here the colicky pain will be associated with vomiting, abdominal distension and obstipation. The cause can be within the lumen of the bowel, within the wall itself or outside. Stricture, bands, adhesions and tumors are some of the common causes for such obstruction. Further details regarding the aetiology of acute intestinal obstruction are beyond the scope of this book. Anyway, diagnosing the exact cause of obstruction is not as important as diagnosing the presence of obstruction itself.
- **Acute enterocolitis:** Acute bacterial or viral infection of the lower gastrointestinal tract will induce spasmodic contractions of the inflamed bowel. Such intestinal colic is usually associated with diarrhoea with or without mucus and blood. History of ingestion of stale food may point towards food poisoning. Needless to say, the foregoing is a non-surgical condition to be managed medically though the patient may present with severe abdominal pain.
- **Ureteric colic:** It is one of the most common causes of severe colicky pain abdomen. Patient will be writhing in pain and demands immediate attention. The fact that the pain is episodic, localised to the flanks ("loin to groin") and often associated with burning micturition as well as haematuria should alert the clinician. Often the pain of ureteric colic is so intense that the patient will not appreciate prolonged clinical examination. If the clinical suspicion of ureteric colic is strong, an antispasmodic

injection will quickly relieve patient's pain thus allowing further examination to proceed.

- **Biliary colic:** This clinical entity is more difficult to appreciate than ureteric colic. For, obstruction of either the cystic duct or the common bile duct is usually associated with localized inflammation thus rendering the pain continuous, though spasm of the biliary tree episodically makes it more severe. There may be associated jaundice, fever, etc. making detection of biliary colic itself more difficult. However a high index of suspicion regarding biliary colic may allow the clinician to detect biliary pathology before the aforementioned complications develop thus benefitting the patient.
- **Uterine contraction:** Uterine contractions can be innocuous (Braxton Hicks contractions); could also be a warning signal for impending abortion or premature delivery. If a pregnant woman presents with colicky lower abdominal pain, always keep the above in mind and do necessary evaluation promptly, e.g. obstetrician's opinion, pelvic ultrasound, etc. before considering acute surgical abdomen. A negative evaluation for an obstetric emergency does not really harm the patient, whereas very minute lost in dealing with an impending abortion will jeopardize both foetal and maternal health.

An easy way to remember the differential diagnosis of acute abdomen is presented below. Again the student is warned that it is more prudent to think of unusual presentation of a common condition than diagnosing a rare disease, when the patient's clinical features are confusing.

- Two most common causes of acute abdomen
    1. Acute appendicitis
    2. Ureteric calculus
- Two acute abdominal conditions which require urgent surgical management.
    1. Perforation of hollow viscus
    2. Acute intestinal obstruction
- Two conditions which require aggressive medical management
    1. Acute pancreatitis
    2. Acute cholecystitis/cholangitis
- Two rare but life-threatening surgical conditions
    1. Mesenteric ischaemia
    2. Aortic dissection/leaking aneurysm
- Two gynaecological causes for acute abdomen
    1. Ruptured ectopic pregnancy
    2. Twisted ovarian cyst
- Two 'medical' causes for acute abdomen
    1. Myocardial ischaemia
    2. Porphyria

The specific symptoms and signs pertaining to each of the above have not been discussed here as it is outside the scope of this book. Some clinical features have been discussed incidentally elsewhere in the book. More details can be had from any good textbook of surgery. However, students would do well to remember that in textbooks the diagnosis is already mentioned before clinical features are discussed, whereas in real life situations we have to recognize the clinical features and based on that reach a plausible diagnosis ourselves. The latter situation is infinitely more difficult than the mere memorization of signs and symptoms pertaining to a specific disease, as is given in textbooks.

Swelling

Swelling is one of the most common reasons for the patient to present himself in the surgical out patient department. Though most of the details regarding a swelling are elucidated during examination, there are a few details which only a patient would know. For example in a large swelling overlying more than one anatomical organ, patient should be asked where the swelling initially appeared. This will give a clue as to the organ of origin.

In evaluating the history of a swelling one should make an effort to find out whether there is any suspicion of malignancy. Rapid growth of the swelling, fungation, loss of appetite as well as weight, evidence of involvement of nearby and/or distant organs are all pointers towards possible malignancy. On the other hand, history of reduction in the size of the swelling can be taken as reasonable evidence that the swelling in question is non-neoplastic.

Students should also keep in mind the essential difference between a swelling and a mass.

A swelling is that which is easily visible to the naked eye. It is essentially a surface lesion. A swelling in the breast is conventionally referred to as a "lump" as it is usually discernible only on palpation. On the other hand, a complex swelling arising from intra-abdominal organs is called a 'mass' so as to differentiate it from a mere swelling or lump. A mass per abdominal can only be appreciated by the doctor using his clinical acumen and not by the patient himself at least in the early stages. An intelligent patient may be able to feel abnormal fullness in some part of his abdomen, but generally the mass has to reach enormous size before the patient himself complains of it. Needless to say, the disease causing it will have reached an advanced stage.

Another aspect of the history of swelling is the possibility of multiple swellings. Patient should be asked if he has any other swelling on his body.

A list of conditions associated with multiple swellings is provided below:

- Multiple, neurofibromatosis (von Recklinghausen's disease of nerves)
- Multiple lipomatosis
- Sebaceous cysts
- Multiple benign lymph nodular swellings caused by conditions like tuberculosis, AIDS, viral fevers, etc.
- Multiple malignant lymph nodular swellings caused by lymphoma, metastatic carcinoma, etc.
- Multiple bony swellings seen in enchondromatosis

Ulcer

An ulcer is perhaps the most common of the surgical symptoms. Like a swelling, an ulcer is also available for easy clinical examination, thus dissuading the student from taking a good history of the symptom. However, even a thorough examination not backed up by good history can remain inconclusive.

One aspect of the ulcer which can not fully or sufficiently be evaluated by examination of the ulcer alone is the presence and character of the discharge. The amount, nature as well as abnormal constituents like bone spicules (in osteomyelitis) or sulphur granules (in actinomycosis) can easily be found out by asking relevant questions to the patient. If the clinical suspicion of a particular condition is high even leading questions can be asked to clarify the situation.

A list of abnormal discharges from an ulcer in provided below:

- Purulent discharge in an infected ulcer
- Scanty serous discharge in a healing ulcer
- Bloody discharge in a malignant ulcer
- Discharge of bony spicules in an osteomyelitic ulcer
- Discharge of "sulfur granules" in an actinomycotic ulcer
- Foul smelling discharge in an ulcer with necrotic debri infected with anaerobic organism.

Vomiting

Vomiting with associated nausea in another common general surgical symptom.

Here one would like to know about the frequency, quantity of vomitus and its contents. Taste and smell of the vomitus can also be a useful guide to the diagnosis. Bitter taste of the bile and sour taste of gastric acid are characteristic.

In inflammatory conditions vomiting is frequent and non-projectile. Here vomiting may be induced by the ingestion of food. But in bowel obstruction the vomiting will be projectile, i.e.

vomitus is literally thrown at a distance and the vomitus might contain undigested food particles eaten the previous day and will be bulky and foul smelling. The vomitus may not contain bile if the obstruction is proximal to the duodenal papilla. The nature of vomitus will change according to the site of obstruction, e.g. bilious vomiting in jejunal obstruction, faeculant vomiting in large bowel obstruction.

Whether or not the vomitus ever contained either altered or fresh blood is another fact to be brought out. Some patients may suppress the history of haematemesis out of fear of a grave diagnosis. This is true especially when they have had only one or two episodes of haematemesis. In a patient who has had at least one bout of haematemesis it is necessary to enquire about melaena or black tarry stools. Though stool may remain black for 3–5 days following a bout of haematemesis, continuing melaena in the face of increasing pallor might suggest continuing internal bleeding.

Regurgitations of food as observed in achalasia cardia and pharyngeal pouch should be differentiated from true vomiting. While in the former the act of regurgitation is passive, effortless and always contains undigested food particles, true vomiting is associated with active reverse peristalsis of the upper gastrointestinal tract leading to epigastric discomfort.

One should always ask whether vomiting is associated with colicky pain or ball rolling sensation in the abdomen. If present, it suggests mechanical obstruction to the gastrointestinal tract. In such cases vomiting relieves the pain, albeit temporarily.

Adynamic obstruction or paralytic ileus may have an extra-abdominal cause like electrolyte imbalance, uraemia, etc. Hence, appropriate history has to be elicited when such is suspected.

It should be borne in mind that vomiting is a highly nonspecific symptom that can be caused by a variety of non-surgical conditions. This probability should be explored if the overall clinical picture does not fit in with any common surgical condition within the abdomen.

Causes for Haematemesis:

- Acute erosive gastritis
- Peptic ulcer-gastric or duodenal
- Oesophageal varices
- Portal gastropathy
- Mallory Weiss tear
- Dieulafoy's lesion
- Carcinoma of the stomach
- Gastrointestinal stromal tumor of upper GI tract
- Iatrogenic—nasogastric tube insertion, endoscopy, anticoagulation, etc.
- Rare causes—Haemobilia, haemosuccus pancreaticus, aorto-duodenal fistula, etc.

Diarrhoea

It is difficult to define what exactly constitutes diarrhoea. Broadly we can say any frequency beyond 3 bowel movements per day or any looseness of consistency constitutes diarrhoea. In the surgical ward one is worried about any recent change in bowel habits rather than long standing functional bowel disturbances.

Colour and quantity of stools are more significant pointers to a surgical pathology than mere increased frequency and loose consistency, e.g. pale colour of the stools in obstructive jaundice; large fatty and foul smelling stools seen in chronic pancreatitis. A detailed list of all the causes of diarrhoea is outside the scope of this book as the list is too long and contains mainly non-surgical causes. However, inflammatory bowel disease and diverticulosis are two of the many such diseases which a surgical resident is called upon to evaluate from time-to-time.

Constipation

Here again the spectrum of normalcy is wide. Hence a recent change in bowel habits is more significant, especially if the symptom is worsening over time and there is history of increasing use of laxatives. In such cases one is likely to be suffering from a surgical pathology like malignancy though there are numerous other causes for constipation.

Causes of constipation:

- Neoplasm
- Stricture
  - Neoplastic
  - Inflammatory
- Colonic pseudo-obstruction
- Hypothyroidism

- Autonomic neuropathy
  - Diabetes mellitus
  - Paraplegia
- Drugs
  - Antidepressant
  - Calcium channel blockers
- Irritable bowel syndrome
- Pelvic floor dysfunction.

Again, the foregoing list contains only the common causes of constipation and is by no means exhaustive.

The variety of causes suggests the need for detailed questioning in relevant cases.

An annoying symptom that accompanies constipation caused by rectosigmoid malignancy is spurious diarrhoea and tenesmus. The very presence of tumour in the region will induce contraction of the rectal musculature with passage of little if any stools, admixed with some blood stained mucus but a feeling of incomplete evacuation persists. Of course, any inflammatory condition affecting the area may also cause similar picture, because of the mucosal irritation that it produces.

The word obstipation or absolute constipation is used when the patient has not passed either stools or flatus over an extended period of time. There is no need to emphasize then that such a patient has intestinal obstruction—either mechanical or adynamic. Other features of obstruction like abdominal distension, pain and vomiting may be associated.

Bleeding Per Rectum

Bleeding per rectum is an important symptom caused by many surgical illnesses. The most common amongst these are haemorrhoids and fissure in ano. But there are many other important causes of bleeding per rectum including colorectal malignancy, ulcerative colitis, angiodysplasia, diverticulosis, etc. which may be missed if proper care is not taken to elicit the details.

Whenever any patient complains of bleeding per rectum one should ask about the duration of the symptoms as well as the frequency of bowel movements. It is worthwhile knowing the colour of the stools as well. Bleeding from the colon will produce bright red blood admixed with stools whereas blood originating from the small bowel is usually altered. Bleeding above the ligament of Trietz produces malaena, i.e black tarry stools. Any associated colicky pain might suggest an inflammatory pathology like dysentery. Rare causes of bleeding per rectum like intussusception produce red currant jelly stools.

Bleeding in classical haemorrhoids is painless, whereas fissure in ano is associated with painful defaecation. One also has to keep in mind the possibility of non-surgical causes of bleeding per rectum like bleeding diathesis, drug induced bleeding, etc.

Causes of lower GI bleeding:

- Anal conditions like piles, polyps and fissure
- Inflammatory bowel diseases like ulcerative colitis and Crohn's disease
- Diverticulosis of the colon

- Colorectal malignancy
- Angiodysplasia
- Meckel's diverticulum, particularly when it contains ectopic gastric mucosa
- Gastrointestinal stromal tumor of the lower GI tract
- 'Medical' causes like enteric fever, rectal varices, dysentery, etc.

As soon as safely possible, after initial resuscitation it is better to arrange for colonoscopy rather than speculate clinically as the patient is usually haemodynamically unstable. Treatment strategy varies vastly depending upon the definitive cause.

Fever

It is a common symptom which accompanies many of the surgical conditions like appendicitis, cholecystitis, cholangitis abscess and even some malignancies. Also one should not forget that a patient in the surgical ward can have or may develop another medical condition as comorbidity. Hence, it is imperative that fever is investigated thoroughly both history wise as well as by lab tests.

Fever can be continuous, remittent or intermittent. Remittent fever shows fluctuation in temperature of more than 2°F but never touches the base line whereas in intermittent fever subsides fully before reappearing. The interval between bouts of fever may vary from hours to days, e.g. malaria.

Fever may be associated with chills and rigors in malaria, abscesses, urinary tract infections, etc. In pneumonitis which is always a threat in postoperative setting, fever will be associated with tachypnoea and breathlessness. Evening rise of temperature is usually a feature of tubercular pathology.

In a surgery ward subcutaneous soft tissue infections, intra-abdominal sepsis, wound infection, etc. are the chief causes for fever. A superficial abscess will show other features of acute inflammation, i.e. redness, swelling and pain. An intra-abdominal pus collection like amoebic or pyogenic liver abscess, perinephric abscesses, subphrenic and pelvic abscesses, appendicular abscess, etc. though more difficult to diagnose can be suspected by the presence of certain associated symptoms,e.g. liver abscess produces pain on jolting movements like climbing stairs. Subphrenic abscess may produce hiccups and pain on deep breathing. Pelvic abscess may produce tenesmus and mucous diarrhoea. Appendicular abscess will be associated with pain in the right iliac fossa. Perinephric abscess will produce pain in the loin as well as urinary symptoms. These symptoms in the appropriate clinical setting should lead the clinician to the diagnosis.

It should be remembered that certain malignancies like renal cell carcinoma, Wilms' tumour, hepatocellular carcinoma do induce fever in the patient. Careless symptomatic treatment of pyrexia in them may lead to disastrous delay in diagnosis.

In the immediate postoperative setting one or two episodes of fever are common and are deemed to be the result of body's reaction to tissue trauma. However, vigilance should be maintained to rule out other causes.

Jaundice

Hyperbilirubinaemia, when it reaches high enough levels becomes noticeable as yellowness of sclera, mucous membranes and finally skin. Occasionally it is the relatives of the patient who will have noticed the jaundice and not the patient himself.

Though jaundice is caused by various viral infections of liver, a student of surgery should be conscious of the fact that jaundice can be due to surgical causes also, e.g. stones obstructing common bile duct, periampullary carcinoma, cholangiocarcinoma, etc. Such obstructive jaundice also produces malabsorption leading to pale and bulky stools. Also patient might have pruritus due to the irritant effect of bile salts on tissue and high coloured urine caused by conjugated bilirubinuria. Periampullary malignancy usually produces progressively deepening jaundice and occasionally haematemesis and melaena along with typical malignant cachexia. There may be a transient waning of jaundice if the tumour tissue sloughs off relieving the obstruction partially. Typically, fever is not a feature unless there is cholangitis, in a case of obstructive jaundice.

Jaundice caused by calculi in the common bile duct is usually associated with colicky pain and fever caused by cholangitis (i.e. Charcot's triad). When a such a patient also has hypotension and mental confusion it is called Reynold's pentad.

For the benefit of students a list of causes for "surgical" or obstructive jaundice is given below:

- *Neoplastic*
  - Cancer head of the pancreas
  - Cholangiocarcinoma
  - Periampullary cancer
  - Cancer of the gallbladder involving the extrahepatic biliary apparatus
  - Metastasis in the lymph nodes at the porta hepatis.

- *Non-neoplastic*
  - Choledocholithiasis
  - Choledochocele
  - Iatrogenic injury
  - Especially during lap cholecystectomy
  - Sclerosing cholangitis
  - Parasites
  - Chronic pancreatitis.

4. What are the factors affecting the symptom?

Many patients report a variation in the severity, character, etc. of a particular symptom brought about by some triggering factor. Some factors might aggravate the symptom while others relieve it, e.g. epigastric pain caused by acute gastric ulcer may be aggravated after food whereas food may relieve pain if the cause is acute duodenal ulcer. Pain of acute pancreatitis, hepatitis, etc. is worsened by jerky movement while the pain in subphrenic abscess aggravates on deep breathing. Claudication pain of peripheral vascular disease is brought about by exercise as well as exposure to cold whereas rest relieves it. Pain of acute sialoadenitis is at its peak during mastication of food. A hernia may become manifest during strenuous exercise and may get reduced on lying down. Also, medicines taken by the patient can affect the symptoms, e.g. epigastric pain of acute gastritis is relieved by antacid tablets. All these factors affecting the symptom will aid the clinician in understanding the pathology underlying symptom.

Factors which affect the character of a symptoms can be listed as below:

- Food or the lack of it
- Medications
- Position of the body
- Physical activity
- Mental status
- Climate

5. How it progressed?

It is vital to follow the progress of any symptom over time. Worsening of symptoms with time might suggest a progression in the pathology and hence the need for diagnosing the condition becomes more urgent, e.g. a swelling which is progressively increasing in size without a decrease in size at any time is more likely to be a neoplasm. Any sudden spurt in the growth of a otherwise slow growing swelling is even more sinister as it may herald the malignant transformation of a benign neoplasm. But one must bear in mind that haemorrhage into a benign swelling might also lead to a sudden increase in the size of the swelling. But in such cases, usually, there may be associated history of trauma, pain, etc.

Some symptoms might change their character over a period of time, e.g. the claudication pain of peripheral vascular disease which comes on only during exercise may become continuous and burning in nature as the disease progresses to involve the nerves. It is then called rest pain. The epigastric pain of acid peptic disease is initially periodic in nature and burning in character. As the disease progresses to produce complications like gastric outlet obstruction, etc. the pain loses its periodicity and becomes dull aching and continuous. On the other hand, symptoms produced by self-limiting conditions or inflammation improve with time, e.g. a resolving haematoma or minor infection.

During the evolution of any disease it is natural that new symptoms might start. It might suggest a complication, e.g. a painless swelling like sebaceous cyst becoming painful on infection. Sometimes it might mean progression of disease, e.g. a duodenal ulcer which initially produces epigastric pain may progress to gastric outlet obstruction leading to projectile vomiting and ball rolling sensation.

6. Any treatment taken? Any tests done?

Another factor that has to be looked into while following the progress of any symptom is whether the patient has had any treatment during the course of the disease. If so, it is worthwhile finding out what specific treatment was given and its effect on the symptom—beneficial or otherwise, e.g. in a case of thyroid enlargement often thyroxine replacement is tried in an effort to suppress TSH production and thereby reduce the size of the gland. T4 replacement is effective in reducing the size of the gland in case of uniform enlargement of thyroid while it may not produce much beneficial effect in a nodular gland. Relevant history needs to be elicited from the patient. Another example of treatment many patients will have tried before presenting in the OPD of a bigger hospital is antiulcer drug therapy for pain abdomen. If the patient has taken the full course of such treatment but still has not derived tangible benefit from it then acid peptic disease is less likely to be the cause of pain abdomen. If any specific investigative procedures like biopsy, FNAC, X-ray, CT, etc. have been done their details should be elicited. This will go a long way in avoiding the repetition of expensive investigative procedures and unnecessary delay in diagnosis and treatment. One should make a mental note to contact the clinician who has treated the patient earlier, if deemed necessary. While one should not be biased by earlier medical opinion, it can be a useful guide as to the probable pathology.

Apart from the foregoing list of questions any other line of questioning that seems relevant and reasonable can be employed by the clinician in an effort to clarify the clinical picture.

Thus, the progress in the patient's symptoms should be traced chronologically from the time he was ill for the first time till the day on which the history is being taken. Often students taking history lose interest in the patient's history beyond the point where patient gets admitted to the hospital. Such an attitude may lead to missing important clues to the diagnosis. It is possible that a patient might have been admitted many days or weeks before the student gets to examine him. Many investigations and therapeutic procedures might have been performed during that time. It is perfectly alright for the student to ask the patient about these procedures and collect the details, if any. It is not the same as seeing the patient's treatment chart and is perfectly acceptable. What the patient can tell you is history proper and can be very useful at times. For example a history of wound debridement in the hospital given by a patient of foot ulcer will go a long way in explaining the regular and punched out edges of the ulcer the student is likely to find later during examination of the ulcer.

CONCLUSION

In this way each symptom that the patient has complained of should be developed so that history becomes more informative. Again students are reminded that details about all individual symptoms have not been included here. This book is only a general planner of history taking and students are advised to refer Textbooks or Clinical Manuals for detailed symptomatology associated with individual organ systems.

4

History on Enquiry

This is necessitated by the fact that a patient may not always give the full history by himself. He will reveal only that information which he thinks is important or relevant. Occasionally he might wilfully suppress some facts as he is either embarrassed or thinks he might offend the doctor. Others might be simply afraid to tell all the details as they think they will be diagnosed to have a major illness if they do so! All of this might lead to inadequate history being taken. These gaps in the history have to be filled by the astute clinician by asking relevant direct and occasionally leading questions. Only then useful conclusions can be drawn from the history.

This process can proceed along three major lines of questioning.

ENQUIRY TO LOOK FOR ANY ASSOCIATED SYMPTOMS

A symptom complained of by the patient will give the clinician a clue as to the probable organ system that is diseased. For example, if a patient complains of epigastric pain it is reasonable to expect that his upper gastrointestinal (GI) tract is diseased though it need not always be so. Diseases of the heart, lungs, lower chest wall, etc. can occasionally produce epigastric pain and discomfort, but in an outpatient setting such causes are much less common than upper GI disorders. Diseases of the upper GI tract may produce a variety of symptoms apart from epigastric pain, like vomiting, flatulence, dyspepsia, retrosternal burning, water brash, jaundice, etc. But the patient may complain of only one, say epigastric pain. This does not necessarily mean the other symptoms are absent. It is for the clinician to diligently coax the history of other associated symptoms if present, from the patient. Only when one knows the full symptomatology can the specific organ involved and the probable pathology can be deduced. In the process of doing this occasionally direct questions may need to be asked. Positive or negative answers obtained for such direct questions are equally important. Students should familiarize themselves with the different symptoms that various disease processes of each organ system can produce. Of course, it is important to remember that pathology of different organ systems can occasionally produce the same symptoms, e.g. myocardial ischaemia is known to cause epigastric pain mimicking acute gastritis; vomiting might be caused GI pathology as well as pathological processes involving brain and inner ear and so on.

ENQUIRY INTO POSSIBLE AETIOLOGICAL FACTORS

The patient may not always know what has caused his ailment. For example, a patient of inguinal hernia may not realize that it is his chronic cough that is the culprit causing the hernia. Occasionally the relationship between a pathology and the symptom it produces may not be apparent. For example, diarrhoea in a patient with thyrotoxicosis. The patient may not know that his neck swelling (thyroid) is the cause of his diarrhoea. It is for the diligent clinician to look for these facts. If these are not found out and properly managed, any symptomatic treatment given for the immediate problem is bound to fail. There is no use prescribing laxatives to a patient who has constipation due to hypothyroidism.

Take for example a case of peripheral vascular disease possibly Buerger's disease. A patient who has come for severe rest pain and blackened toe may not be aware that it is his smoking that is doing the damage. Here it is justifiable to discuss his smoking habit within presenting history itself rather than keeping it till personal history is asked as smoking is a major aetiological factor for peripheral vascular insufficiency. After all there is a difference between smoking by a patient of peripheral vascular disease and a patient of lipoma doing so. By discussing smoking in presenting history itself, student can convey the importance attached to it by him.

Similarly for different possible pathological conditions, aetiological factors either in the patient's lifestyle, occupation or in other co-morbid conditions like diabetes mellitus, tuberculosis, hypertension, etc. should be looked for and recorded if present. Here student should use his common sense and restrict himself to enquiring about commonly found causes for the most probable condition that the patient might have. Otherwise, since at this stage of history, diagnosis is still in doubt the list of such questions can be endless. Also it is here that language skills are most needed. Unless the query in the clinician's mind can be translated into a simple question that the patient can easily understand and respond to, the whole exercise is likely to be futile. Do always remember that the patients are not likely to know medical terminology. Hence, it is worthwhile knowing the regional language translations of most commonly asked questions. Of course the ultimate effort should be to acquire a working knowledge of the language itself.

Another point that I would like to emphasize here is that one should never entertain very rare diagnosis. It has been rightly said "You will be rarely correct if you make a rare diagnosis". It is always safer to think of atypical presentations of a common condition when one encounters an unusual case.

Yet another thing to remember is that tuberculosis is always a candidate in the differential diagnosis of almost any disease. Unfortunately this is the bitter truth in our country, even today. Hence, it is always wise to enquire about history of contact with tuberculosis and any other fact which might suggest its possibility.

Finally one may round off this part of history by asking the patient for history which might reveal that he is diabetic, hypertensive or asthmatic. Very often there is a tendency to relegate these things to the past history. Asking for it while discussing presenting history itself is justifiable on two counts. One is that all these are major comorbid conditions which may directly or indirectly be involved in the causation of the presenting symptoms. Second, these diseases being not completely curable, sadly never become "past history". Once an unfortunate patient has them, he has them for life! If the patient has any of such conditions then details about the treatment that the patient is taking should be sought and recorded.

ENQUIRY INTO POSSIBLE COMPLICATIONS

A pathological process affecting any organ might become manifest in differing degrees of severity. Sometimes a patient suffering from a particular disease may develop a complication which might need a different strategy if diagnosed. These differing degrees of severity of the pathology as well as complications might produce specific symptoms which when recognised will aid in diagnosis. A typical example is a thyroid swelling. Patient may complain of only a neck swelling but it is up to the clinician to find out from the patient whether he might have symptoms suggestive of malfunctioning of the gland or even malignancy. Loss of weight inspite of increased appetite, heat intolerance, excessive sweating, palpitation, diarrhoea, etc. are some of the symptoms that suggest the diagnosis of thyroid hyperfunction. Lethargy, weight gain, loss of hair, constipation, etc. might suggest hypofunction. Hoarseness of voice, dysphagia, dyspnoea, point to either malignancy or pressure on the larynx and so on.

Students are encouraged to think of possible complications, given patient's history, and ask question accordingly. But it is necessary that the line of thinking is logical and should relate to a pathology probable in the patient in view of his history.

It is this clinical 'enquiry' that fleshes out the history and makes it meaningful. The gaps in the history are thus filled and there is better perception of the patient's condition. Otherwise history taking becomes a monotonous exercise devoid of any creativity. Such dry and questionnaire based history is likely to be of limited use.

Also such intimate questioning actually reassures the patient that the clinician is genuinely interested in his welfare.

5

Past History (Including Medical History)

There is tendency amongst students to breeze through past history once they are through with history of presenting complaints. At best a history of similar episodes in the past is all that is sought to be elicited. "Past history is not contributory" or "No relevant past history" are commonly heard dismissive phrases in the clinical class. Well, such lopsided approach is what makes the history taken useless.

To begin with let us be clear about what constitutes past history. If refers to a point of time in the patient's past which is separated from the presenting history by period of normalcy. The patient will have enjoyed a period of apparently normal health till presenting complaints start. A typical example would be recurrent acute appendicitis. Sometimes an attack of acute appendicitis resolves completely on conservative management only to recur months later. In between the attacks the patient might have had no symptoms. Here the earlier attack becomes part of past history. Similar episodes may be present in the past history of patients suffering from ureteric colic, acute pancreatitis, etc. On the other hand, if the patient was never completely alright following the first attack then the whole history starting from the first attack should be considered presenting history, e.g. chronic pancreatitis, ulcerative colitis irritable bowel syndrome, etc.

It is important to realize that past history may have other significant medical or surgical details. Any major illness that the patient may have suffered in the past, especially that for which patient was hospitalised should be recorded. One may find some such episode might directly or indirectly be connected with the current illness. For example, suppose a patient with presenting complaints of leg ulcer gives history of having been bedridden in the past for a period of time due to any illness. It is possible that the deep vein thrombosis that the patient might have had at that time is the factor behind the venous ulcer that the patient has now! Another famous example is a patient who has had resectional surgery on a body part in the past and now presents with a swelling elsewhere. Here the possibility that the previous surgery was done for a malignant condition should always be kept in mind. Otherwise we might end up unnecessarily investigating the cause of metastatic swelling for which the patient has presented. Therefore accurate history as regards amputation if any done in the past should be obtained.

Similarly, all the surgical procedures that the patient has ever had with the type of anaesthesia used should be recorded. Any surgery has its own long-term complications which might predispose to patient's current troubles, e.g. An appendicectomy operation might damage the ilioinguinal nerve leading to weakening of abdominal wall and direct inguinal hernia. A laparotomy might induce peritoneal adhesions which may cause pain abdomen. Even if the previous surgery is not contributing to the current illness it will give information regarding patient's surgical fitness and thus about comorbid conditions, if any. In any case student will have demonstrated his diligence in history taking by recording such facts about the patient's past.

Also in past history, information regarding any drug allergy or adverse reaction that the patient might have had should be sought. This might mean the difference between life and death for an occasional patient. If such history is present then the fact should be recorded in bold letters and also entered on the front sheet of case file.

History regarding physical as well as mental health milestones and immunisation might be needed occasionally, especially in a paediatric patient.

Thus, a well taken past history can provide useful information which might shed light on the aetiology of current set of symptoms, besides directing further examinations.

6

Occupational History

Many occupations have associated physical hazards. For example, traffic policemen have to stand for long periods of time, construction workers run the risk of fall from heights, factory workers face the risk of accidents, etc. But one should not be under the impression that it is only the physical aspect of an occupation that can lead to ill health. Any job can be associated with mental stress in addition to physical strain. Even amongst people doing white collared jobs psychosomatic ailments are common and often have their origin in job related stress, lack of rest and relaxation, etc. In today's hectic world, job related stress is having its ill effects on marital life too thus jeopardizing health further. And of course the nature of work often determines patient's financial status which in turn determines utilisation of health care facilities. For example, it is unlikely that a manual labourer will be rich and so on.

The students taking occupational history should routinely record the nature of work and whether or not work involves physical strain. An effort should be made to look for any work related factor which might have contributed to patients ill health either mental or physical, like long hours of work, working in shifts, lack of job security, etc.

There are some popular beliefs amongst students about certain occupations causing certain specific disease. These are not necessarily true. Like bus drivers being susceptible to acid peptic disease. Such preconceived notions should be abandoned. Then there are certain occupational diseases like chimney sweeper's cancer, etc. which are too rare to be of much practical significance.

The following is a list of common occupations with their associated health hazards. These hazards might cause ill-health by themselves or may aggravate a preexisting disease process. The list is by no means exhaustive. The students are encouraged to add to the list.

Occupation	*Health hazards*
1. Agriculturist	• Poor economic status • Walking bare feet in wet surroundings • Poor access to medical facilities • Lack of education • Traditional beliefs • Pneumoconiosis
2. Manual labourer	• Poor economic status • Having to lift heavy objects • Prone for minor injuries
3. Salaried office worker	• Work related mental stress • Lack of physical exercise • Malingering to avail medical leave
4. Employee in software industry	• Lack of rest • changing work schedule and expectation • Job related stress • Postural problems due to working long hours on a computer

Contd...

Contd...

Occupation	*Health hazards*
5. Factory worker	• Factory accidents • Irregular working hours due to working in shifts • Noise pollution
6. Truck driver	• Road traffic accidents • Easy access to cheap sex • Irregular food habits • Alcoholism
7. House wife	• Domestic accidents like scalds, cuts • Over work, especially in joint families • Marital discords and lack of self respect • Attention seeking due to lack of appreciation for work at home
8. Unemployed	• Poverty • Low self esteem leading to drug addictions

A treatment strategy planned for the patient should take into account his occupation as well as economic status. A change of occupation may have to be advised occasionally as a last resort if his current occupation is deemed to be contributing to his illness.

7

Personal History

It is always necessary to gain insight into the kind of person that the patient is because many of the illnesses have their origin in the lifestyle and habits of the patient. On the other hand, the disease itself might affect patient's lifestyle. For example, if a postman were to have peripheral vascular disease he will find it difficult to do his job.

It is necessary to collect personal details of the patient discreetly without offending him. It is better not to be judgemental in these matters. Accordingly one should not use words like 'alcoholic' 'chronic smoker', etc. in describing habits. It is enough if one restricts oneself to describing facts. For example one can say "patient smokes about 20 beedies per day and has been smoking for the last 10 years. "Patient consumes about 100 ml of whisky 2–3 times per week" and so on. Drug addiction in any other form like tobacco chewing, narcotic abuse, etc. should also be noted down.

Next, one has to enquire about patients diet-whether vegetarian or mixed. The word 'non-vegetarian' should be avoided as its meaning is ambiguous. Again an effort should be made to look for anything in the patient's dietary habits which might have contributed to his illness. A dramatic example of this is the tropical pancreatitis that is endemic in parts of Kerala where diet includes large amounts of tapioca. Excessive ingestion of hot and spicy food might contribute to acid peptic disease. Many colonic diseases are linked to diet.

Most illnesses usually affect appetite in an adverse way, e.g. chronic diseases like tuberculosis, malignancy, etc. usually lead to loss of appetite and consequent loss of weight. But some disease processes might actually improve appetite, e.g. thyrotoxicosis, diabetes mellitus, etc. In thyrotoxicosis there is loss of weight in spite of increased appetite. In diabetes mellitus there is associated polydipsia and polyuria. Students should learn to differentiate loss of appetite from early satiety. Appetite is the desire to ingest food in an effort to alleviate hunger. Early satiety means patient's hunger is satisfied with small amounts of food though the patient might initially have the desire to have food. Another confusing situation is when the patient is reluctant to eat in spite of having adequate appetite as ingestion of food exacerbates symptoms, e.g. gastric ulcer, chronic pancreatitis, etc.

Bowel and bladder habits of the patients also should be routinely recorded. Most pathological conditions of the gastrointestinal tract affect bowel motility. There are many non-gastrointestinal conditions too which might also affect bowel movement, e.g. thyroid dysfunction, diabetes, drugs, etc. Any recent change in the bowel or bladder habits is more significant as it may herald disease process. Alternatively, poor bowel and bladder training itself may be the cause of patients illness. For example, chronic straining at stool or micturition can be a causative factor for hernia, piles, rectal prolapse, etc. Use or misuse of laxatives should be asked about if the patient has long standing constipation. Increased frequency of urine at night might suggest incomplete bladder evacuation as is commonly the case in benign prostatic hypertrophy.

Whether or not sleep is affected is another matter to be enquired into. Sleep disorder may be the cause or effect of many ailments. A patient who is deprived of proper sleep is distressed, irritable and looks sick. The cause for sleeplessness should be sought. It might be due to the severity of his physical symptoms or due to some other stress. Many factors like fear of death, poverty, sick family members, etc. might make the patient anxious and thus result in lack of sleep. Any history of regular use of sleeping pills is significant. On the other hand, if a patient says his sleep is not disturbed then it is likely that is symptoms are not of severe nature. It is worthwhile to remember that there is hardly any disease conditions which induces sound and restful sleep!

Menstrual history has been discussed separately.

8

Family History

This is another important area which does not receive the attention it deserves while recording history. Many a time "no significant family history" is all that one gets hear from he student presenting the case. Let us first tell ourselves what we are looking for in the family history.

Many diseases run in families due to genetic predisposition. Multiple neurofibromatosis (von Recklinghausen's disease of nerves) and haemophilia are the classical examples. Diabetes mellitus is perhaps the most common example. Essential hypertension also runs in families. But more dramatic is the familial association of certain cancers, e.g. carcinoma of the breast.

Genetic predisposition need not be the only reason why an illness affects many members of a family. Sometimes close social contact that family members have is all that is required for a communicable disease to affect many members of the same family. Tuberculosis is one such scourge affecting mostly poorer sections of our society. Alternatively, an endemic disease might affect more than one member of a family, as also others in the neighbourhood, e.g. Iodine deficiency goitre, malaria. And finally if the disease process is the result of malnutrition one can expect more than one member of the family to be affected similarly.

One should always enquire about similar illness amongst close relatives. Death amongst first degree relatives (parents and siblings) should be recorded and reasons sought.

It is not out of place here to enquire about any marital disharmony. Problems between husband and wife or between any two members of a family may be the root cause for many physical symptoms that either of them might develop later. Many so called psychosomatic illness have their origin in such emotional stress. A compassionate clinician might be able to inspire enough confidence in the patient that he may reveal these very personal and intimate facts to him. Without such skills at counselling one is bound face frustrating failures in treating such patients.

A well taken family history gives the clinician a holistic view of the problem at hand. Many a time unless the problem is tackled at a similarly holistic level, mere treatment of resultant symptoms is doomed to fail.

The socioeconomic class to which the family of the patient belongs often contributes to the causation of the disease and occasionally determines the kind of treatment that can be offered.

It is interesting to note that it is not only poverty that contributes to illness but also affluence. Obesity, diabetes, cardiovascular problems, etc. are more common among the affluent class than rest of the society.

9

Menstrual History

This part of the history tends to get neglected especially in an emergency room setting. In their anxiety to arrive at a quick diagnosis, students or some times even senior consultants fail to elicit detailed menstrual history. This might lead to the disastrous overlooking of early pregnancy and subjecting the mother as well as foetus to battery of harmful investigations including exposure to X-rays and drugs. Do make it a habit to ask about at least the date of last menstrual period in every case where the patient is a female in the reproductive age group if you want to avoid such a catastrophe and of course litigation. In case of unmarried women one has to be tactful in eliciting history which might suggest pregnancy, without offending the patient or parents. Any case of secondary amenorrhoea should be considered as pregnancy unless proved otherwise by pregnancy tests and ultrasound.

The details about menstrual history should include the age at menarche, the regularity and duration of menstrual cycles, amount of flow, any abnormal flow, age at menopause, etc. Date of last menstrual period has to be recorded routinely so as to avoid the problems discussed earlier. If the patient is taking oral contraceptive pills, it should be noted. A brief obstetric history should be taken.

Past history of caesarean section if present, should be recorded. History of intrauterine contraceptive device (IUCD) placement or tubal ligation should be sought and noted, if present.

Of course, any association between the current symptoms and the menstruation should be looked for, e.g. painful breast nodule of fibroadenosis becomes more painful during menstrual flow. Endometriosis is another condition which produces symptoms during menstrual periods.

In a general surgical setting the significance of menstrual history is in ruling out early pregnancy. Patients are not likely to volunteer information about menstrual cycles unless it forms part of their presenting complaint. It is up to the clinician to elicit that history before proceeding to examine the patient and asking for investigations.

Gynaecological symptoms like white discharge, dysmenorrhoea, dysfunctional uterine bleeding, etc. should be recorded if present but further evaluation often needs a gynaecologist's guidance.

10

Do's and Don'ts in the Surgery Ward

Do report on time for the ward rounds.

Do conduct yourself in a dignified manner. It is expected of you by patients. It is difficult for a patient to entrust his health care to a shabbily dressed and giggling youngster.

Do sympathize with the patient; after all he is the one who is sick and suffering and not you. He can be irritable, irrational or uncooperative.

He may even get angry. Put yourself his position and you will understand him better.

Do smile at patients. Obviously, they would not want their doctor also to look gloomy. A smile costs you nothing and increases your face value.

Do respect patient's privacy. Imagine how you would feel if stripped near naked in front of curious onlookers.

Do carry a clinical manual and a note book. The manual will help you to refresh your clinical skills and the note book to jot down any pearl of wisdom you might come across.

Do wash your hands before and after examining each patient.

Do ask for help when you feel you need it. Do not wait till the patient feels you need help.

Do respect the nursing staff. It is likely they will have spent more years in the surgical ward than you. Occasionally, they may even be able to guide you.

Do wear your white coat and carry your own stethoscope, measuring tape, pen torch and other necessary paraphernalia.

Do discuss with your colleagues about cases which you think unusual or complicated.

Do fill the requisition forms for investigations correctly.

Do take informed consent before any invasive procedure.

Do learn the local language.

Do believe in God.

Don't examine any patient without his consent.

Don't lose your temper with any patient, however, badly he might have behaved.

Don't expect the patient to be intelligent and wise always. In fact a dumb or foolish patient needs you even more.

Don't examine a female patient without a lady attendant or staff sister being in attendance.

Don't strip a patient without providing adequate privacy.

Don't examine a patient without explaining to the patient what it involves. Imagine how you would feel if a dozen people suddenly descend on you and start squeezing your tummy.

Don't leave a wound open after you have finished examining it.

Don't wake a patient from sound sleep unless it is really necessary.

Don't ever feel that the patient has come merely to trouble you. Patients come because they are suffering and not to trouble some unknown doctor. Even a malingerer has a problem, albeit psychological.

Don't expect your diagnosis to be correct all the time; It is your analytical and logical approach to a clinical problem that is to be developed. Diagnostic accuracy will definitely improve with time if your approach is right.

Don't discuss the poor prognosis of a disease arbitrarily in front of the patient.

Don't be impatient with patient's relatives. They have reason to be anxious. If properly approached they can provide useful information regarding patient's illness.

Don't take shortcuts during ward work. It may cost the patient his life and you your job.

Don't argue with your seniors.

Don't go to the ward if you yourself have a communicable infection.

Don't discriminate between patients based on social status, religion, caste, etc.

Don't leave the paper work incomplete.

Don't look down on patient's with HIV infection whatever be the cause of infection.

11

Points to Ponder

Think of the following while working in the ward.

- Patient is the centre of the medical universe.
- Eyes do not see what the brain does not know.
- It is better to read and fail than fail to read!
- People do not care how much you know, until they know how much you care.
- And finally, like somebody once said "Once I had the blues,
  Because I had no shoes.
  Until upon the street.
  I met a man who had no feet."
  Try and help the less fortunate and you will enjoy the satisfaction and sense of fulfilment that it gives you.

12

Model Case History

What follows is a model for taking history in a patient with thyroid problem. I would not say this is the only way to take history or that this history cannot be bettered. In fact I am sure anybody can take an equally good or better history provided the desire to do so is there.

Mr Ramappa walks into the surgeon's consulting room looking anxious and scared. The good doctor had already noticed the personal details entered in the empty case file placed in front of him by the OPD nurse. So he addresses the patient straight away by name "come on, Mr Ramappa, take your seat. Please do tell me how I can help you." Ramappa who was apprehensive till then immediately felt relaxed and sits across the table and starts narrating the story. Here is how the conversation went (Needless to say adequate privacy has been ensured).

Mr Ramappa : Doctor I am having this swelling in front of my neck

Doctor : Since when?

Mr Ramappa : For the last 1 year

Doctor : Do you have any other complaints?

Mr Ramappa : Nothing in particular that I can think of. Why doctor, what am I having?

Doctor : Let's see. Tell me the whole story from the beginning. You Told me it started 1 year ago. How did it start?

Mr Ramappa : I don't know. About a year back my friend noticed the swelling and told me. It was very small at that time not more than pea size. See now it has slowly grown into the size of lemon.

Doctor : Did you have any pain in the swelling anytime?

Mr Ramappa : No

Doctor : Have you been to a doctor during this time?

Mr Ramappa : I did, 6 months ago

Doctor : What was done then?

Mr Ramappa : The doctor advised me to get a needle test done. He also said I needed some blood tests.

Doctor : Did you get those done?

Mr Ramappa : No sir, I did not get the needle test done as I was afraid. But my blood test was found normal. I was told I have a thyroid swelling.

Doctor : Oh I see, Do you have any change in voice, breathlessness, difficulty in swallowing, etc. after the onset of this swelling? (Looking for pressure symptoms and /or infiltration).

Mr Ramappa : No

Doctor : Do you, feel lethargic, fatigued all the time? Have you been putting on weight recently? What about bowel movements? (Looking for evidence of hypothyroidism).

Mr Ramappa : No doctor, I do not feel any different now compared to one year ago.

Doctor : Do you feel sweaty, feverish all the time? Has your appetite improved in recent days? (Looking for features suggestive of hyperthyroidism).

Mr Ramappa : No. Like I already told you I do not feel any different.

Doctor : Have you been taking any medication?

Mr Ramappa : Yes. I am taking 2 tablets daily. One was given for this swelling by the earlier doctor. I take it everyday early in the morning but the swelling has not come down one bit. The other tablet is for the control of BP. I forgot to tell you. I have been taking this tablet for the last 4 years. But otherwise I am fine. No diabetes, no heart problem.

Doctor : That is good. Show me those tablets during your next visit. (Doctor expects one of the drugs to be eltroxin being given in an attempt to reduce the size of the thyroid). By the way, do you have any other swelling in the neck? (Wants to rule out lymph nodular enlargement).

Mr Ramappa : As a matter of fact yes, I did notice a small swelling on the side of the neck one week ago. I thought it is not important. Why do you ask?

Doctor : Just like that, do not worry. I will explain after I have examined you. Now tell me, does any of your family members or neighbours have similar complaints?

Mr Ramappa : I do not think so. But then, I am not sure about all neighbours.

Doctor : That is okay, have you undergone any surgeries before ? Where you admitted at any time?

Mr Ramappa : Never

Doctor : Do you smoke or drink?

Mr Ramappa : I have never consumed alcohol in my life. I used to smoke but now I have stopped.

Doctor : Since when?

Mr Ramappa : For the last 6 months

Doctor : That is good. Any problem you have as regards sleep, bowel and bladder function?

Mr Ramappa : Nothing in particular.

Doctor : What is your normal diet?

Mr Ramappa : I am a vegetarian.

Doctor : Do you like cabbage a lot?

Mr Ramappa : No, actually I hate cabbage. What is the connection with my problem anyway?

Doctor : Well, eating a lot of cabbage can cause thyroid gland swelling in the neck in some people. Anyway it does not apply to you. So do not worry.

Mr Ramappa : What is my problem, doctor. Is it serious?

Doctor : It appears to be an enlargement of thyroid gland called goiter. Let me examine you thoroughly and then come to further conclusion.

Doctor then proceeds to examine the patient and advises regarding further line of management.

13

Impediments to Good History Taking

This chapter has been added in this edition, so as to summarise the potential problems in communicating with the patient. In today's world, where society no longer believes in "doctor knows best" policy, the best safeguard against allegations of medical negligence is proper communication.

How to communicate well with the patient has been described in detail in this book. However just being knowledgeable about the process does not necessarily mean good history is being taken all the time. There can be many impediments to it. Some of the common impediments have been listed below. It is interesting to note that, not all of them can be remedied by the clinician alone. Active participation by the patient as well as facilitation by the hospital management is equally important if history taking has to flourish. Let us now discuss in brief the impediments.

POOR COMMUNICATION SKILLS ON THE PART OF THE CLINICIAN

- *Language barrier:* Without a working knowledge of the local language useful communication is impossible. At least local language translations of commonly asked sentences should be known to students if they hope to make their history taking exercise worthwhile.

- *Cultural bias:* It is possible that the student belongs to an entirely different social class, caste or religion. He or she may be from a region far away from the place where the hospital stands. It is possible that the student may even be from another country. All these can lead to cultural bias wherein the student may not appreciate the social norms, customs, lifestyle, etc. leading to inadequate questioning. However with effort it is possible to overcome these barriers.
- *Gender barrier:* In a conservative society like ours it is possible that the student is not comfortable interacting with patients of opposite sex, especially if they are young. The fear of being misunderstood also adds to the discomfort. As long as one maintains a strictly professional attitude, explaining the need for questioning in a clear but polite way, it should be possible to get used to this situation within a short time.

POOR COMMUNICATION FROM PATIENT'S SIDE

- *All of the above:* It goes without saying that whatever areas of discomfort that the student has in discussing health problems with the patient, the same things trouble the patient too. A patient who is sick may not even have the mental strength to overcome these barriers.
- *Fear:* Hospital is an intimidating place for most people, leave alone patients. Once within the hospital premises patient begins to worry about his disease condition, prognosis, cost of

treatment, possible surgery, etc. A worried mind is not always rational. Hence the history given may not be the best one possible under circumstances. It is left to the astute clinician to make the patient reassured and comfortable before starting the process of history taking.

- *Poor intellect:* Always remember that patients need not be an intellectual or wise person. Some patients may not have the intellectual capacity to clearly elucidate their symptoms. A few of them may actually be mentally challenged. A clinician should take it as a challenge to interact with such patients so that as much useful information as is possible is gained from the interaction.

  It is sometimes seen that mentally challenged people as well as innocent kids give the best history as their responses are not colored by mental stress.

- *Poor physical state:* It goes without saying that an acutely sick patient will not be in the mood for a lengthy conversation. His mind and memory may not be clear. Hence a more pro-active strategy has to be employed, wherein only the absolutely necessary aspects of history are elicited and further examination of the patient commenced.

  This strategy is most applicable in the emergency room where undue delay is not advisable in the management of severely ill or trauma patients. However, once the patient's health stabilises more information may be forthcoming either from the patient or from the attendants.

- *Psychiatric illnesses:* A patient of psychiatric illness presenting with a surgical condition can be a tricky challenge. Whereas the patient may not be able to give a coherent history, the clinician will tend take whatever the patient says with disbelief. While the assistance of the relatives is invaluable under such circumstances, a more understanding and perseverant approach may be needed to get the correct picture from the patient himself. For example, no relative can say whether the pain felt by the patient is in the right iliac fossa or otherwise. Only the patient himself can do that.

POOR INFRASTRUCTURE AND WORKING CONDITION

Many a time neither the doctor nor the patient can be blamed for the poor communication. If a doctor is expected to see hundreds of patients everyday it will be impossible for him to do a good job of communicating with his patients. This kind of situation exists in many busy general hospitals where each consultation lasts barely a couple of minutes.

On other hand, even if the doctor or student has the time, if the infrastructure is poor, good history taking becomes impossible. Adequate privacy is a must. Consulting rooms must be well lit and reasonably furnished. In the wards, students must ensure that patients are not left insulted, intimidated or embarrassed by insensitive questioning in front of curious onlookers.

The above paragraphs should make it clear that not all impediments to a good history taking can be overcome by the clinician all by himself. Indeed, it is a teamwork between the doctor, institution and of course the patient.

14

Conclusion

I am sure you will have realized by now that the aim of this book is not to replace existing clinical manuals but to augment their value. An effort has been made to encourage the students of surgery to empathise with the patient, communicate effectively with him and finally understand him and his illness. This understanding when coupled with clinical and theory knowledge and common sense will lead to the correct diagnosis in most cases. Of course, as has already been said, it is an art which will take a life time to perfect. But it is worth pursuing. And rewarding too.

Once again let me assure you that no advance in technology will replace the clinician. If anything, rational use of technology needs even better understanding of clinical aspect of the pathology. And the satisfaction of having been able to help a patient by merely employing better communicative skills is reward enough for your effort. No equipment, however, state of the art it may be, can infuse the kind of confidence in a patient that a sympathetic clinician can.

Well, I have put in my effort. If this books helps at least a few students of clinical surgery in understanding their patients better I will consider my effort worthwhile.

Index

A

B

C

D

E